62 Healthy survival foods

Dr. Lucy Coleman

COLEMAN PUBLISHING

Coleman Publishing

62 healthy survival foods

A guide on sustainable healthy foods for emergency situations

Dr. Lucy Coleman

www.LifeBossNetwork.com

Contents

Introduction

The urgency of preparedness

Emergencies. Crises. Pandemics. Natural disasters. Lockdowns. Wars.

These words carry with them a heavy burden—fear, panic, uncertainty, and the sudden disruption of life as we know it. Yet, amid the chaos, one word echoes above all others: survival.

Survival is not just about making it through the storm; it's about maintaining your strength, health, and resilience when the world around you is changing in unimaginable ways. And at the core of survival lies a fundamental truth: you cannot survive without food.

We often prepare for emergencies by thinking about shelter, medicine, power sources, or personal safety—but too frequently, food is an afterthought. This oversight can lead to devastating consequences. Even in the safest shelter, without the proper nourishment, your body becomes weak, your immune system falters, and your ability to think clearly or act decisively is compromised.

This book was written to shift that mindset.

In moments of disaster, access to healthy, nutritious food becomes limited. Supermarket shelves are emptied. Supply chains are disrupted. Safe cooking or refrigeration may no longer be possible. The best way to protect yourself and your family is to prepare in advance—stocking your home with survival foods that are shelf-stable, nutrient-dense, and capable of sustaining your health in the toughest conditions.

Through this guide, you'll discover practical strategies for building a smart food storage plan that focuses not just on calories—but on immunity, energy, and wellness. You'll also learn how to make your own survival foods, such as homemade energy bars, and how to eat for strength and clarity when food becomes scarce.

Inside, you'll find:

- A practical roadmap to emergency nutrition

- The top 62 survival foods to store and how to use them

- Guidelines on food storage, shelf life, and preservation

- Tips for maintaining energy, immunity, and mental clarity

- Simple, homemade recipes for nourishing meals in tough times

Each chapter is designed to be clear, actionable, and adaptable to different lifestyles and dietary needs. Chapters 3, 6, 7, 8, and 9 are dedicated to breaking down the full list of 62 essential survival foods into categories—making it easier to build your pantry and tailor it to your family's needs.

Whether you are preparing for a short-term emergency, a long-term crisis, or simply want peace of mind, this book will serve as your essential survival food guide.

Let's begin this journey by exploring how to master emergency nutrition—because when disaster strikes, the time to prepare is already over.

Chapter 1

How to get the best out of emergency nutrition

Emergencies—whether triggered by natural disasters, pandemics, wars, or economic collapse—have one thing in common: they disrupt access to essential resources. Among these, food is paramount. During such times, nutrition becomes not just a matter of health, but survival. This chapter lays the foundation for everything you'll learn in this book, offering key strategies to help you stay nourished, resilient, and energized during uncertain times.

1. Stockpile the right foods

The first step in emergency nutrition is strategic preparation. It's not enough to fill your pantry with whatever is available. Choosing the right kinds of food can make the difference between staying healthy and falling into nutritional decline.

Imagine being locked down at home with only sugary cereals, processed snacks, and soda. These might satisfy short-term cravings but will weaken your immune system and energy levels over time. Instead, prioritize nutrient-dense, shelf-stable foods like beans, lentils, oats, whole grains, nuts, seeds, canned fish, and dehydrated vegetables. These provide the macronutrients (protein, healthy fats, and complex carbs) and micronutrients (vitamins and minerals) your body needs to thrive.

This book contains carefully curated lists of 62 survival foods divided into practical categories to help you build a well-balanced, health-supporting emergency pantry. Use them to start preparing now—before crisis strikes.

2. Embrace homemade nutrition

Chapter Three of this book will guide you through making your own energy bars and high-protein snacks using simple ingredients. The ability to create nutritious, long-lasting food at home gives you independence and control during emergencies.

In many crisis situations, store-bought foods become scarce or unaffordable. Rather than stressing over what's unavailable, learn to make your own replacements. You'll find that with a few key ingredients—like oats, honey, seeds, and dried fruits—you can prepare power-packed snacks that fuel your body and strengthen your immune system.

Homemade food is not only cost-effective but also free of preservatives and artificial additives. In survival scenarios, your body deserves real, clean food.

3. Grow your own garden

Even a small garden can make a significant difference. Whether it's a full vegetable patch, raised beds, or a series of potted herbs on a balcony, homegrown produce ensures a fresh supply of vitamins and antioxidants, even when store shelves are empty.

Gardening connects you to the source of your food and builds resilience. Leafy greens, tomatoes, sweet potatoes, carrots, and medicinal herbs like garlic or ginger can be grown in most climates with a little planning. You'll not only save money but also gain peace of mind knowing that you can feed your family no matter the circumstances.

4. Understand your unique nutritional needs

Emergency food planning isn't one-size-fits-all. Your individual health profile should influence what you store and consume. If you have chronic conditions like diabetes, high blood pressure, or food allergies, be mindful of how your emergency food stock supports—or hinders—your health.

It's also wise to consider the needs of children, the elderly, or pregnant individuals in your household. Tailoring your food supply to suit these specific needs ensures that everyone stays nourished and well-supported.

In non-crisis times, take the opportunity to identify nutritional deficiencies and adjust your pantry accordingly. A personalized approach makes all the difference when food access becomes limited.

5. Use this book's detailed survival food lists

Each chapter of this book is designed to help you take immediate action. The 62 survival foods are broken down into practical categories for energy, immunity, digestion, mood, and long-term storage.

These lists are more than suggestions—they're a blueprint. They offer variety, nutrient density, and versatility, so you can plan well-rounded meals no matter how long the emergency lasts. If you ever feel overwhelmed, just start with one category and gradually expand.

Nutrition is the most overlooked pillar of survival. This book empowers you to fix that by focusing on real, powerful foods that will carry you through the toughest situations.

In summary

Survival begins with preparation, and preparation begins with food. This chapter has introduced you to the key strategies you need to create an emergency nutrition plan that supports your body and your health:

- Choose the right foods, not just the available ones.

- Learn to cook your own nutritious meals and snacks.

- Grow what you can, even if it's just herbs on a windowsill.

- Consider your family's unique nutritional needs.

- Use this book's food lists as a step-by-step guide.

In the next chapter, we'll dive deeper into specific vitamins and minerals that are crucial during times of crisis, and how to ensure your body gets them even when fresh food is scarce.

Let's turn fear into preparedness and panic into empowerment—starting with what's on your plate.

Chapter 2

Getting the most out of fiber, protein, carbohydrates, fats, vitamins, and minerals

I n times of crisis, your body becomes your most valuable asset. Fueling it properly with essential nutrients—especially fiber, protein, carbohydrates, healthy fats, vitamins, and minerals—can make the difference between barely surviving and staying strong and resilient.

This chapter dives into the practical strategies you can use to get the most from these key nutrients using emergency-ready foods. Whether you're relying on shelf-stable items or limited fresh produce, understanding how to combine and prioritize your food sources is the first step in maintaining immune strength, energy, and physical performance when it matters most.

Fiber: The forgotten hero of digestion

Fiber supports digestion, keeps bowel movements regular, and promotes a healthy gut microbiome—an essential part of the immune system. During an emergency, it also keeps you feeling fuller longer, which is especially helpful when rations are limited.

Best practices to maximize fiber intake:
- Choose whole fruits over juices to retain the fiber content.

- Snack on high-fiber options like dried figs, dates, and trail mix with seeds.

- Prioritize legumes, canned beans, and whole grains (e.g., brown rice, oats, quinoa).

- If baking, use high-fiber flours such as coconut, chickpea, or barley flour.

- Consider fiber supplements (like psyllium husk) if fresh produce is scarce, but only under medical supervision.

Protein: Building immunity and strength

Protein is vital for muscle repair, immune function, and cell regeneration. In emergency settings, it's easy to rely on carbs alone, but protein-rich foods will sustain your strength and help you fight off illness.

Tips to boost protein intake:

- Eat protein-rich items first in your meal (e.g., tuna, eggs, or jerky) to optimize nutrient absorption.

- Add protein sources to every meal: canned chicken or fish, nut butters, powdered protein shakes.

- Use plant-based proteins like lentils, black beans, and canned chickpeas when meat is limited.

- Store shelf-stable protein powders for quick, nutritious shakes.

Carbohydrates: Energy to power through

Carbs often get a bad reputation, but they are a critical fuel source—especially during physically or emotionally draining periods. The goal is to focus on complex carbohydrates rather than processed ones.

Smart carbohydrate choices:

- Stock whole grains like oats, brown rice, and quinoa.

- Include legumes and starchy vegetables like canned sweet potatoes or lentils.

- Limit refined carbs, sugary snacks, and processed baked goods.

- Balance your meals with fiber and protein to reduce blood sugar spikes.

Healthy fats: Fueling brain and body

Fats are necessary for hormone production, cognitive function, and nutrient absorption. They help regulate inflammation and keep you feeling satisfied between meals.

How to optimize fat intake in emergencies:

- Choose heart-healthy fats like olive oil, coconut oil, and avocado oil for cooking.

- Snack on nuts, seeds, or nut butters.

- Include canned fatty fish like sardines, mackerel, or salmon.

- Add flaxseed or chia seeds to oatmeal or smoothies for an omega-3 boost.

Remember, moderation is key—fats are calorie-dense, so small portions go a long way.

Vitamins and minerals: The micronutrient backbone

Your immune system can't function without a steady supply of vitamins and minerals, especially vitamins A, C, D, E, and B-complex, as well as zinc, magnesium, calcium, and iron.

Maximize nutrient retention:

- Steam or lightly cook vegetables rather than boiling them to preserve nutrients.

- Grill or bake meats instead of frying.

- Include canned and frozen fruits and vegetables to maintain variety.

- Mix different types of produce to hit your "5 servings a day" target, even when using shelf-stable options.

- Take a multivitamin if food access becomes too limited (consult a healthcare provider if possible).

Pro Tip: Keep dried herbs and spices on hand—parsley, oregano, turmeric, cinnamon—not only for flavor but also for their potent antioxidant and anti-inflammatory properties.

A final note on bioavailability and balance

No single food has everything your body needs. To get the best from your emergency nutrition, aim for variety and balance. Combining certain foods helps improve nutrient absorption. For example:

- Pair vitamin C-rich foods (like canned bell peppers or citrus) with plant-based iron sources (like lentils) to boost absorption.

- Include healthy fats (like olive oil) when eating fat-soluble vitamins (A, D, E, and K) for better uptake.

- Drink plenty of water to help fiber do its job properly and aid digestion.

What's next?

Now that you understand how these six essential nutrient groups work together for optimal survival health, it's time to move into practice.

In Chapter Three, you'll learn how to prepare five homemade energy bars packed with the protein, fiber, and micronutrients your body craves during a crisis.

These recipes are simple, customizable, and most importantly—shelf-stable and life-sustaining.

Let's get started!

Chapter 3

5 healthy homemade energy bars and the process of drying food for emergencies

Energy bars are a good source of energy for individuals because of their high nutritional content that includes cereals and other high energy foods. Energy bars are a great example of the kind of foods to have in storage for an emergency because, in addition to being vitamin and minerals fortified, they can last a while.

While you may not trust some energy bars produced by food companies because they can expire quickly, you do have the option of making your own bars at home. Healthy homemade energy bars can be made, eaten, and remade for the duration of the emergency.

If you have kids during such emergencies, you will also need to have healthy snacks at home, and energy bars are an excellent alternative to sugar-dense snacks.

So in this chapter, you will learn how to make five easy energy bars at home. You will also unearth the basic concepts of drying foods as a healthy food preservative measure.

We will begin how to make five energy bars at home:

Energy bar 1

Ingredients:
- Seedless dates

- Dried cranberries

- Dried cherries

- Almonds

- Pistachios

- All ingredients above should be in equal proportion.

Steps:
- Combine all ingredients in a food processor and process until they all break and form a solid mass.

- Roll the softball mass between butter papers into a thick square and refrigerate for 30 minutes.

- After 30 minutes, bring out the mix and with a pizza cutter (or a sharp knife), outline bar lines.

- Cut out each bar and store.

- Your homemade energy bar is ready!

Energy bar 2

Ingredients:
- 1 cup nuts (your preferred nut choice)

- Cup dried fruit

- 1 cup pitted dried dates

Steps:
- Roast nuts or use them in their raw form (the roasting is optional), but if you roast, it will add some more toasty flavour to the bars.

- If you roast, then do it at 350F for 10-12 minutes until they are fragrant and golden. Set aside to cool before taking the next step.

- Mix the nuts, dried fruits, and dates in a food processor and pulse a few times to break them up. Always pause the processor to separate dates that clump together.

- Process for an additional 2 minutes while scraping the edges of the bowl to prevent some of the mix sticking to it.

- Continue with the processor until a ball is formed.

- Lay on a piece of wax paper on a work surface and press the dough with your hands until you form a square.

- Chill in the refrigerator overnight

- The following morning cut out bars from the dough and start eating! The remaining bars can be stored in the fridge.

Energy bar 3

Ingredients:

- 1 cup almond butter (other nut butter of your choice is okay)

- 1 cup almonds (roughly chopped or pulsed)

- 1 ½ cup of uncooked oats

- ½ cup honey (you can use maple syrup)

- 2tbsp coconut oil

- 1.2 salt (optional)

- For mix-ins, you will need dried tart cherries, chocolate chips, or other dried fruits and nuts.

Steps:

- Combine the almonds, cranberries, mix-ins, and oats.

- Heat honey, coconut oil and nut butter on low heat and pour into the oat and almond mix then stir together.

- Transfer to an 8x8 inch dish and flatten into a square.

- Cover the bowl and refrigerate overnight.

- The following day cut them in squares and store.

- Enjoy your healthy energy bar!

Energy bar 4

Ingredients:
- 1 cup nuts

- 1tbsp vanilla extract

- ¼ cup honey

- ½ cup peanut butter

- Nutmeg (a pinch)

- 1/2 tsp ground cinnamon

- 2tbsp chia seeds

- ½ cup raisins

- 1 cup oats

Steps:
- Using a bowl or large food processor pulse nuts until thoroughly ground.

- Add raisins, chia seeds, cinnamon, nutmeg, and oats, then pulse for 1 second to combine.

- Add peanut butter, vanilla, and honey, pulse all ingredients one last time.

- Scrape the mix into an 8x8 baking dish, press firmly and evenly then refrigerate for two hours or until it is firm.

- Use a knife to slice bars out of the mix and enjoy your bar!

Energy bar 5

Ingredients:

- 1 cup dry oatmeal

- ½ cup peanut butter

- 2/3 cup toasted coconut flakes

- ½ cup flax seeds (ground)

- 1tbsp chia seeds (optional)

- 1tsp vanilla extract

- 1/3 cup honey (or agave nectar)

- ¼ cup cocoa powder (unsweetened)

Steps:

- Combine and mix ingredients in a medium bowl.

- Cover the pan and refrigerate its content for at least half an hour

- After it's chilled, cut into bars and store in airtight bags in the refrigerator overnight.

- Your bars are ready!

The concept of drying food for emergencies

Drying is a way of food preservation, and it is also known as dehydration. When foods are dried, moisture is reduced, thus eliminating bacteria growth that aids deterioration of food. There are different means of drying food that includes:

Oven drying

Oven drying works with oven trays where the food is placed on and the oven set at the lowest (not below 140-150 degrees). As the food dries up in the oven, moisture will escape, and the food will be free from bacterial.

Sun drying

Sun drying is one of the oldest means of drying food, and it is also a natural means of keeping food safe for a long time. All fruits and foods should be placed under direct sunlight, and you can repeat the same process with the same food for about three days until you get the dried texture.

Dehydrator

Dehydrators are in two forms: solar and electric. Just decide on the type you want and follow the manufacturer's manual.

Below you will find a shortlist of some specific vegetables you can dry during survival period and things to note about the process. Most of the methods below also apply to fruits, but we are using vegetables because they are important immune boosters during emergencies. Note that these are a few vegetables to illustrate the point you can dry as many other vegetables as you want.

Carrots

- Wash carrots and cut off roots

- Peel and cut into slices or strips at 1/8 inch thick

- Dry until it is tough

Asparagus

- Wash properly and halve in large parts

- Dry until it is leathery to brittle

Broccoli

- Trim and cut (as though you want to serve it)

- Wash the stalks and dry until it is crisp and brittle

Green beans
- Wash and cut into pieces

- Dry until it is very brittle

- Store for future use

Tomatoes
- Steam tomatoes in boiling water to loosen the skin

- Chill in cold water

- Peel the skin and slice ½ thick or cut into ¾ sections.

- Dry until its crisp and store.

Spinach
- To dry spinach, first, trim the leaves and wash them.

- Shake or pat dry them then remove excess moisture.

- Dry for about two minutes until crisp and store.

With energy bars and dried foods at home, you can survive any emergency or sudden frightening experiences at home because these are superfoods and easy methods of staying healthy. During health emergencies such as a virus outbreak, you must ensure that your immune system is strong enough to handle the crises. Also I the case of a natural emergency that might leave you trapped for a while, and you might need all of your energy to escape as soon as it is safe for you and your family. Next, we will discuss how to boost your immune system with survival foods.

Chapter 4

Homemade energy bars & food drying: Two lifelines for emergency nutrition

W hen emergencies strike, having nutrient-dense, energy-boosting foods at your fingertips can make the difference between vulnerability and strength. Energy bars are compact, convenient, and power-packed sources of essential nutrients—making them ideal survival foods. Unlike processed snack bars full of sugars, preservatives, and artificial ingredients, homemade energy bars allow you to control what goes into your body, ensuring both nourishment and longevity.

This chapter serves two critical purposes:

1. Teach you how to make five easy, nutritious, and delicious energy bars at home.

2. Introduce the principles of food drying—a traditional and highly effective method for preserving fresh produce without refrigeration.

Whether you're preparing for a power outage, natural disaster, pandemic, or isolation period, these methods will help you stock your pantry with reliable, healthy options that support your immune system and keep your energy up.

Section One:

5 Homemade energy bar recipes

These energy bars are made with shelf-stable ingredients, don't require baking, and are ideal for children and adults alike during stressful times.

Energy bar #1: Cherry-pistachio delight

Ingredients:

- Equal parts: Seedless dates, dried cranberries, dried cherries, almonds, and pistachios.

Instructions:

- Pulse all ingredients in a food processor until a sticky mass forms.

- Roll into a thick square between sheets of parchment paper.

- Refrigerate for 30 minutes.

- Cut into bars and store in an airtight container.

Energy bar #2: Nut & fruit fusion

Ingredients:

- 1 cup mixed nuts (almonds, cashews, etc.)

- 1 cup pitted dates

- 1 cup dried fruit (apricots, raisins, or figs)

Instructions:

- Lightly roast the nuts at 350°F for 10–12 minutes if desired.

- Pulse all ingredients in a food processor until a sticky dough forms.

- Press into a square on wax paper and refrigerate overnight.

- Cut into bars and store.

Energy bar #3: Oats & almond butter squares

Ingredients:

- 1½ cups oats

- 1 cup almond butter

- ½ cup honey or maple syrup

- 1 cup almonds (chopped)

- 2 tbsp coconut oil

- Optional: dried cherries, chocolate chips, or dried fruit

Instructions:

- Combine dry ingredients.

- Warm almond butter, honey, and oil in a saucepan.

- Mix together and press into a dish.

- Refrigerate overnight and cut into bars.

Energy bar #4: Cinnamon raisin chia bars

Ingredients:

- 1 cup nuts

- ½ cup oats

- ½ cup raisins

- 2 tbsp chia seeds

- ¼ cup honey

- ½ cup peanut butter

- ½ tsp cinnamon, a pinch of nutmeg

- 1 tbsp vanilla extract

Instructions:
- Grind nuts, then pulse all dry ingredients.

- Add wet ingredients and pulse again.

- Press into a baking dish, chill for 2 hours, and slice.

Energy Bar #5: Chocolate coconut protein bars

Ingredients:
- 1 cup oats

- 2/3 cup toasted coconut flakes

- ½ cup peanut butter

- ½ cup ground flaxseeds

- 1 tbsp chia seeds

- 1 tsp vanilla extract

- 1/3 cup honey or agave

- ¼ cup unsweetened cocoa powder

Instructions:
- Mix all ingredients in a bowl.

- Chill for 30 minutes.

- Cut and store in airtight bags.

Section Two: The art of food drying for long-term storage

When refrigeration is not available, drying food is one of the most effective preservation strategies. Dehydrating removes moisture, preventing the growth of bacteria and mold while concentrating flavor and nutrients.

Drying methods:

1. Oven drying
   - Set oven to the lowest setting (140–150°F).

   - Spread food thinly on baking trays.

   - Leave the oven door slightly open to let moisture escape.

   - Turn food periodically for even drying.

2. Sun drying
   - Place thin slices of fruit or vegetables on mesh screens in direct sunlight.

   - Cover with cheesecloth to protect from insects.

   - Bring indoors at night.

   - Repeat for 2–3 days until leathery or brittle.

3. Electric or solar dehydrators
   - These are more efficient and adjustable than traditional methods.

   - Follow the device's specific settings for different types of food.

Quick guide: How to dry common vegetables

Carrots
   - Wash, peel, and slice into 1/8-inch strips.

   - Dry until leathery and store in airtight jars.

Asparagus

- Wash and cut large spears in half.

- Dry until leathery or brittle.

Broccoli

- Cut into small florets, blanch briefly, and dry until crisp.

Green Beans

- Cut into 1-inch pieces.

- Dry until completely brittle.

Tomatoes

- Blanch, peel, and slice.

- Dry until crisp (for sun-drying, it may take several days).

Spinach

- Wash and dry the leaves.

- Dehydrate until fully crisp.

Why this matters

Energy bars and dried foods are more than just backup meals—they are functional tools in your emergency nutrition kit. They are portable, nutrient-rich, and long-lasting, giving you the confidence that no matter the crisis, you have food that fuels, heals, and strengthens.

When prepared in advance, these options empower you to stay calm and resilient—even in the face of uncertainty. In the next chapter, we'll explore how survival foods can actively support and boost your immune system.

Chapter 5

When disaster strikes

How to manage and consume your emergency foods wisely

H aving a well-stocked pantry filled with nutritious emergency foods is a powerful first step—but survival isn't just about what you have. It's about how you use it. When a disaster hits, panic and uncertainty can lead to poor food decisions, overconsumption, or even waste. This chapter is designed to help you prepare mentally and practically for that moment, ensuring your hard work in building a stockpile truly serves its purpose.

In this chapter, we go beyond what to eat and focus on how to eat—strategically, mindfully, and resourcefully. These are the key actions that will help you make the most of your survival foods and maintain your physical and emotional strength throughout any emergency.

1. Plan your meals thoughtfully

When times are uncertain, structure becomes your lifeline. Planning your meals ensures balanced nutrition and helps prevent mindless eating driven by stress or boredom. It also allows you to stretch your supplies over time, avoiding the risk of running out early in the emergency period.

Tips:

- Create a flexible weekly menu using available ingredients.

- Focus on nutrient-dense meals with protein, fiber, and healthy fats.

- Alternate between shelf-stable and perishable items early on to avoid spoilage.

2. Establish regular meal times

During a crisis, normalcy is soothing. Maintaining regular mealtimes provides psychological stability and keeps your metabolism functioning well. It also ensures that food is shared fairly among household members, especially children.

Tips:

- Set consistent breakfast, lunch, and dinner hours.

- Incorporate small snack breaks if necessary.

- Use timers or a written meal schedule on the fridge to keep everyone on track.

3. Snack smart—no exceptions

In stressful times, sugary or salty snacks may seem comforting, but they offer little value to your immune system or energy levels. If your pantry is filled only with healthy choices, your body—and your mind—will thank you.

Smart snack ideas:

- Homemade energy bars from Chapter 3

- Dried fruit, roasted chickpeas, nuts, or whole-grain crackers

- Freeze-dried veggie chips, apple slices with peanut butter, or dark chocolate in moderation

4. Motivate healthy eating— even when morale is low

Disasters can drain your emotional resilience. Boredom, fear, and anxiety often lead to emotional eating or cravings for unhealthy comfort food. If you have children, they will be especially vulnerable to this behavior.

Strategies:

- Make healthy eating a fun, family-based activity—prepare meals together.

- Create colorful plates with dried or canned veggies, fruits, and protein sources.

- Celebrate small health wins like staying hydrated or trying a new food combination.

5. Monitor inventory with a simple tracking system

Keeping a visual or written log of what you have helps you manage portions, reduce waste, and avoid surprises. During an emergency, it's easy to forget how much has been used and how much remains.

Suggestions:

- Use a notebook or whiteboard to track food quantities and expiration dates.

- Prioritize foods nearing expiration.

- Divide portions into daily or weekly rations if resources are limited.

6. Waste nothing— every bite counts

Even during non-crisis times, food waste is a major issue. During emergencies, it's unacceptable. Teach everyone in your household that every meal matters. Just because you prepared extra doesn't mean it should be discarded.

Waste - reduction ideas:

- Use vegetable peels in homemade broths.

- Turn stale bread into croutons or breadcrumbs.

- Store leftovers in airtight containers, clearly labeled for later use.

7. Be generous when you can— share with purpose

One of the most meaningful acts during an emergency is sharing. There may be neighbors, elderly people, or low-income families who were unable to prepare. If you have the means to spare a few items, you can make a life-changing difference.

Ways to share responsibly:

- Set aside a small portion of your pantry for charitable giving.

- Partner with community relief efforts or local shelters.

- Share foods that are nutrient-dense, easy to prepare, and shelf-stable.

Final thoughts: From storage to strength

This chapter is not just about food consumption; it's about intention. Emergencies bring out both the best and worst in us. Your preparation isn't complete until you know how to manage your resources with wisdom, discipline, and compassion.

Let this chapter serve as your practical and emotional guide to making your food last, keeping your body nourished, and ensuring that no effort you've made toward survival goes to waste.

In the next chapter, we'll explore the foods and nutrients that directly support your immune system—and why a strong immune response may be your most vital asset during any crisis.

Chapter 6

8 Survival superfoods that aid digestion and strengthen the immune system

When facing a crisis or natural disaster, it's not just about having food to eat—it's about having the right food to keep your body functioning optimally. Two of the most essential pillars of health during emergencies are digestion and immunity. Poor digestion can leave you bloated, uncomfortable, and sluggish, while a weakened immune system can increase your risk of illness—especially in stressful, unsanitary, or isolated conditions.

In this chapter, we focus on eight science-backed superfoods and supplements that support both digestion and immune function. These foods are not only shelf-stable or easy to store but also potent allies for staying healthy when access to fresh food or medical care may be limited.

Why digestion and immunity matter in emergencies

During emergencies, your routines change drastically. You may be more sedentary, under stress, dehydrated, or consuming foods you don't normally eat. These changes can strain your digestive system and suppress your immune function. Choosing the right foods helps:

- Maintain regular bowel movements

- Prevent nutrient malabsorption

- Reduce inflammation and oxidative stress

- Support your gut microbiome

- Help your body defend against viruses, bacteria, and environmental stressors

Here are eight powerful superfoods and supplements to include in your emergency nutrition plan:

1. Raw Honey

A natural sweetener and medicinal food with an infinite shelf life, raw honey is much more than just a sugar alternative. Rich in antioxidants, it helps reduce blood pressure, ease digestive discomfort, and regulate blood sugar. Its antimicrobial properties can also soothe sore throats and suppress coughs.

Survival benefits:

- Long-lasting and doesn't spoil

- Soothes gastrointestinal issues

- Can be used topically for minor cuts and burns

- Supports immune function naturally

2. Digestive enzymes (from whole foods or supplements)

Digestive enzymes break down the food we eat into absorbable nutrients. In survival scenarios, eating unfamiliar or less varied foods may cause indigestion or bloating. Enzymes assist your body in digesting fats, proteins, and carbohydrates efficiently.

Natural sources:

- Pineapple (bromelain)

- Papaya (papain)

- Mango, banana, kiwi, avocado, and raw honey

Tip: You can also store high-quality digestive enzyme capsules to supplement meals during high-stress times or when eating heavy foods.

3. Apple Cider Vinegar (ACV)

A time-tested home remedy, ACV supports digestion by increasing stomach acid and promoting healthy gut bacteria. It also helps stabilize blood sugar and reduce cholesterol.

Suggested use: Mix 1 tbsp with warm water and a little honey before meals to stimulate digestion.

Additional benefits:

- Helps relieve indigestion and bloating

- Supports immune health

- May reduce sugar cravings

4. Green Tea

Packed with antioxidants called polyphenols, green tea is one of the healthiest beverages to keep in your emergency pantry. It reduces inflammation, enhances digestion, and supports immune response at the cellular level.

How to enjoy:

- Brew hot or cold

- Combine with lemon or ginger for added benefits

- Store both loose-leaf or bagged for flexibility

5. Fiber powder (PsylliumHusk, Bran, etc.)

Fiber is essential in any diet, but especially in low-activity settings like lockdowns or shelter-in-place scenarios. It keeps bowel movements regular, helps detoxify the body, and promotes feelings of fullness, reducing unnecessary snacking.

Forms to store:

- Psyllium husk powder

- Ground flaxseed

- Bran or methylcellulose powders

Bonus: Fiber also feeds your beneficial gut bacteria, supporting long-term immune health.

6. Vitamin C powder (or whole food sources)

Vitamin C is a foundational immune-boosting nutrient. In powder form, it stores well, is easy to dose, and is free from unnecessary additives. It enhances white blood cell function, supports wound healing, and acts as a powerful antioxidant.

Best forms:

- Pure ascorbic acid powder

- Camu Camu powder (one of the most vitamin C–dense foods)

- Whole fruits like oranges, lemons, kiwis, and strawberries when available

7. Fish oil (or Omega-3–rich fish)

Omega-3 fatty acids help reduce inflammation, regulate immunity, and support cardiovascular and brain health—critical factors during high-stress times.

Best sources:

- Canned or frozen fish: salmon, mackerel, sardines, tuna

- Fish oil capsules (check expiration dates and store in a cool place)

Pro tip: Buy fish packed in olive oil for double the nutritional benefit.

8. Water Kefir grains

Water kefir is a probiotic-rich fermented drink that improves gut health and enhances immune defense. Unlike dairy-based kefir, water kefir is vegan, shelf-stable (in dried form), and can be brewed at home using just sugar water and kefir grains.

Health benefits:

- Improves gut microbiome

- Reduces inflammation

- Provides hydration with added benefits

How to make:
- Use filtered water, organic cane sugar, and dried kefir grains

- Ferment at room temperature for 24–48 hours

- Flavor with fruit or ginger for taste

Final thoughts

The superfoods covered in this chapter are not just functional—they are foundational. They help maintain digestive comfort, support nutrient absorption, and power your immune system through the stress and uncertainty of a crisis.

By integrating these into your emergency pantry or survival food kit, you'll ensure your body has the tools it needs to stay resilient—both physically and mentally. Keep in mind that consistency matters: it's not about eating them once, but using them regularly throughout your emergency preparedness and recovery plan.

Next, we'll take a deeper dive into the broader topic of nutrition strategies in survival scenarios—how to combine food groups, time your meals, and stay nourished when resources are limited.

Chapter 7

11 Survival foods to boost nutrition

When preparing for emergencies, it's easy to focus on calories and quantity—but true preparedness also means focusing on quality. Nutrient-dense foods that are rich in vitamins, minerals, antioxidants, and essential fatty acids are the cornerstone of maintaining your energy, mental clarity, immune function, and digestive health during times of stress and limited access to fresh food.

This chapter highlights 11 survival superfoods that not only store well but also deliver concentrated nutrition. These foods can be easily added to your pantry or emergency kit, ensuring your body continues to receive what it needs to thrive, not just survive.

1. Wheat germ

Wheat germ is the most nutrient-rich part of the wheat kernel. It's an excellent source of folate, magnesium, zinc, potassium, and vitamin E, making it a powerful antioxidant food.

How to use:

- Sprinkle on oatmeal, yogurt, or smoothies

- Mix into baking recipes or energy bars

- Use as a breadcrumb substitute for extra nutrition

Benefits:

- Boosts the immune system

- Supports heart health and red blood cell production

- Enhances digestion and nutrient absorption

Storage tip: Keep in the refrigerator or freezer to preserve freshness and avoid rancidity.

2. Chlorella

Chlorella is a freshwater green algae packed with chlorophyll, protein, B vitamins, and iron. It's a detoxifying superfood known to bind heavy metals and boost immune response.

How to use:

- Add 1 tsp to smoothies or juices

- Take in tablet or powder form

Benefits:

- Supports detoxification and gut health

- Enhances immune system performance

- Helps regulate blood sugar and blood pressure

3. Spirulina

Another algae powerhouse, spirulina is rich in protein, iron, antioxidants, and essential amino acids. It has anti-inflammatory effects and can help combat fatigue, stress, and anemia.

How to use:

- Stir into smoothies or juices

- Add to soups or energy bars

- Mix with water and lemon for a nutrient shot

Benefits:

- Natural energy booster

- Supports immune regulation

- Enhances red blood cell production

4. Protein powder

Protein is an essential macronutrient, especially important in situations where you may be less physically active or eating irregular meals. Choose plant-based or whey protein depending on your dietary preference.

How to use:

- Blend with water or non-dairy milk

- Add to oatmeal, pancakes, or baked goods

- Use post-exercise to aid recovery

Benefits:

- Preserves muscle mass

- Supports tissue repair and hormone production

- Provides a satisfying and stable energy source

5. Multivitamins

A well-rounded multivitamin ensures you're covering potential gaps in your emergency diet. Even with good food choices, vitamin and mineral intake can drop when access to fresh produce is limited.

Tip: Look for a high-quality multivitamin with active forms of B vitamins, vitamin D3, and minerals like selenium and zinc.

Benefits:

- Improves energy levels

- Supports mental clarity and immune health

- Helps maintain metabolic balance

6. Liquid minerals

Unlike tablets, liquid mineral supplements offer better bioavailability and faster absorption. They are especially useful when digestion is compromised, or when hydration and electrolyte balance are priorities.

Popular types:
- Magnesium

- Potassium

- Trace minerals blends

Benefits:
- Relieves fatigue and muscle cramps

- Supports nerve and heart function

- Helps manage stress response

7. Flax seeds

Flax seeds are rich in omega-3 fatty acids, fiber, and lignans, offering powerful anti-inflammatory and hormone-balancing benefits.

How to use:
- Add to smoothies, oatmeal, or baked goods

- Use as an egg substitute in recipes

- Grind before eating for optimal absorption

Benefits:
- Supports heart health

- Improves bowel regularity

- Helps regulate cholesterol

Storage tip: Store whole seeds in a cool, dark place. Grind as needed.

8. Eggs

Eggs are one of the most complete foods—rich in protein, vitamin D, choline, and selenium. If stored properly, they can last for 2–3 months in a refrigerator under 55°F. Coating them in mineral oil can further extend shelf life.

Benefits:

- Versatile for cooking: breakfast, snacks, or baked meals

- Excellent protein source for kids and adults

- Supports brain function and immune strength

9. Coconut oil

Coconut oil is shelf-stable and incredibly versatile. It contains medium-chain triglycerides (MCTs) that are quickly converted to energy, supporting metabolism and brain function.

How to use:

- For cooking, baking, or raw treats

- In teas, smoothies, or as a natural energy boost

- Externally for skin and wound care

Benefits:

- Antibacterial and antifungal properties

- Supports liver and digestive health

- Helps stabilize blood sugar

10. Chia Seeds

These tiny seeds pack a punch—loaded with omega-3s, protein, fiber, and antioxidants. They absorb up to 12x their weight in liquid, making them ideal for hydration and satiety.

How to use:

- Add to smoothies, yogurt, or energy bars

- Make chia pudding

- Sprinkle on top of cereal or salads

Benefits:

- Supports digestive health and hydration

- Stabilizes blood sugar

- Promotes heart and joint health

11. Cacao powder

Unlike processed cocoa, raw cacao powder is rich in flavonoids, magnesium, iron, and antioxidants. It can elevate mood, support cardiovascular health, and reduce inflammation.

How to use:

- Mix into smoothies or protein shakes

- Use in baking or homemade hot chocolate

- Sprinkle on oatmeal or fruit bowls

Benefits:

- Boosts serotonin and dopamine levels

- Protects heart and brain

- A natural mood and energy enhancer

Final thoughts

Nutrition is the cornerstone of resilience. In times of crisis, the body and mind are under stress, and proper nourishment is one of the few things you can control. These 11 survival superfoods will help you maintain strength, focus, and immunity—no matter how long the emergency lasts.

They're easy to store, versatile to use, and powerful in their nutritional profile. Begin adding them gradually to your pantry today so you're ready, not reactive.

In the next chapter, we'll look at bulk survival foods—those long-lasting staples you should stock up on in quantity to prepare for the long haul.

Chapter 8

11 Bulk food items to stockpile for long-term emergencies

Stockpiling is a foundational pillar of emergency preparedness. When done wisely, it ensures your family has access to nutritious, versatile, and long-lasting foods—without the chaos of last-minute panic buying. It's important to distinguish between thoughtful stockpiling and reactionary hoarding.

Panic buying occurs when people suddenly realize they're unprepared and rush to stores during or just before a crisis. This often leads to:

- Overbuying perishable or unhealthy items

- Overspending on non-essential foods

- Missing out on key ingredients that support health and variety

By contrast, strategic stockpiling is planned, purposeful, and built gradually. It ensures you have the essentials on hand for meals that are nutritious, comforting, and easy to prepare even under stress.

In this chapter, we'll explore 11 key bulk food items to keep in your emergency pantry. These foods are long-lasting, widely available, and flexible enough to support a range of dishes—from breakfasts to snacks to hearty meals.

1. White and brown rice

Rice is a universal survival staple. It's calorie-dense, shelf-stable, and incredibly versatile.

- White rice lasts longer (up to 25–30 years when stored properly).

- Brown rice has more fiber and nutrients but a shorter shelf life (6 months to 1 year).

Use it for: stir-fries, soups, casseroles, grain bowls, or breakfast porridge.Storage tip: Store in airtight containers or vacuum-sealed bags in a cool, dry place.

2. Spaghetti and other pasta

Pasta is affordable, easy to store, and quick to prepare. It pairs with everything—from simple tomato sauce to more complex stews and stir-fries.

Go for: whole-grain or legume-based pasta for extra fiber and protein.Tip: Practice portion control to balance carbohydrate intake.

3. Potato flakes

Instead of instant mashed potatoes loaded with additives, consider making your own homemade potato flakes by dehydrating thinly sliced potatoes.

Nutritional value: Rich in fiber, potassium, vitamin B6, and vitamin C.Use them: as a thickener for soups, a side dish, or even in baking for moisture.

4. Pancake mix or ingredients

Pancakes offer comfort and versatility. Stock a healthy pancake mix, or better yet, keep core ingredients like oats, flour, baking powder, and milk powder.

Add-ins: dried fruits, cinnamon, seeds, or powdered protein.Bonus: Pancakes can be adapted for savory meals too!

5. Oats

Oats are a nutritional powerhouse—high in fiber, protein, and essential minerals.

Use them for:
- Breakfast porridge

- Homemade energy bars (see Chapter Three)

- Baked goods and granola

- Meatloaf or veggie burger filler

Preferred type: Traditional rolled oats store longer and have better texture than instant oats.

6. Non-fat dry milk

Milk is useful for baking, cooking, and drinking—but during emergencies, refrigeration may be limited. Non-fat dry milk is an ideal substitute.

Use in: coffee, pancakes, smoothies, soups, sauces, and baked goods. Storage tip: Store in airtight containers and keep away from humidity.

7. Macaroni and small pasta shapes

Macaroni and other small pasta types like elbow, penne, or orzo are excellent for soups, casseroles, pasta salads, or one-pot meals. Their short cooking time also makes them energy-efficient in a crisis.

Tip: Pair with canned beans, veggies, or a spoonful of coconut oil for a full meal.

8. Granola

Granola is more than a breakfast—it's a portable, no-cook snack rich in healthy fats, fiber, and protein. Choose options with nuts, seeds, and dried fruit or make your own for better control over sugar content.

Uses:

- Eaten on its own

- Topped over yogurt or rehydrated milk

- Stirred into nut butters or baked goods

9. Cocoa mix or cacao powder

A morale-booster in hard times, cocoa mix or cacao powder brings warmth and a touch of indulgence.

Cacao powder is rich in antioxidants and beneficial minerals like magnesium and iron. Use it for:

- Hot chocolate

- Smoothies

- Baking

- Homemade energy snacks

Choose unsweetened cacao powder for the healthiest option and sweeten it naturally with honey or dates.

10. Berry drink mix or freeze-dried berries

Berries are packed with antioxidants and vitamin C—but they spoil quickly. A berry drink mix, especially one free of artificial sweeteners, is a convenient way to enjoy their benefits.

Alternatively, stock up on freeze-dried or frozen berries to blend into drinks or mix into oatmeal, pancakes, and trail mixes.

11. Beans (dry or canned)

Beans are one of the best survival foods you can buy. They're rich in fiber, protein, and essential minerals, and incredibly shelf-stable.

Stock varieties such as:

- Black beans

- Pinto beans

- Chickpeas

- Kidney beans

- Great northern beans

Tips:

- Dry beans store longer, but canned beans are quicker to prepare.

- Rinse canned beans to reduce sodium levels.

- Use beans in soups, rice dishes, dips, stews, or even baked goods (like black bean brownies).

Final thoughts on stockpiling

Stockpiling doesn't mean hoarding—it means preparing with intention and balance. These 11 foods provide a strong base for endless meal combinations that will keep you nourished, satisfied, and healthy during difficult times.

Here's what makes these foods ideal: Long shelf life Nutritional density Versatility in recipes Easy to store and rotate

By choosing your bulk items wisely, you'll be able to build meals that are not only filling but also support your immune system, digestion, energy levels, and mood.

In the next and final chapter, you'll find a comprehensive survival grocery list that combines all the foods and strategies we've covered so far—so you can build your pantry with confidence.

Shall we continue to Chapter Nine: The ultimate survival grocery list?

Chapter NineEssential grocery list: 35 foods for long-term storage

When preparing for an emergency, having a well-thought-out grocery list is key to maintaining health, nutrition, and variety in your meals. This chapter contains a comprehensive guide to the most important food staples that can be stored long-term, allowing you to feed your family nourishing meals—even during extended disruptions.

Food storage is not about hoarding; it's about mindful preparation. These items are shelf-stable, nutrient-rich, and highly versatile—allowing you to create healthy meals, snacks, and beverages without depending on frequent grocery trips.

Use this list when stocking up or rotating your pantry to ensure you're always ready.

1. Sweetened powdered drink mix

Choose mixes sweetened with natural options like stevia, monk fruit, or erythritol. These are useful for hydration and flavor without harmful additives.

2. Seeds

Flax, chia, hemp, sesame, sunflower, pumpkin, and even watermelon seeds are packed with fiber, minerals, and healthy fats. They're perfect for smoothies, bars, or baking.

3. Herbs & spices

Essential for flavor and health. Stock up on turmeric, garlic powder, black pepper, cumin, oregano, basil, rosemary, thyme, dill, onion powder, smoked paprika, cayenne, and cinnamon. Dried herbs last for years when kept airtight.

4. Pretzels (low-sodium)

A fun, crunchy snack with long shelf life. Choose whole wheat, low-sodium versions if available.

5. Healthy pre-mixed canned drinks

Look for drinks fortified with electrolytes or vitamins (e.g., coconut water, vitamin waters) without added sugars.

6. Potato chips (baked or homemade)

Buy air-dried or baked chips with minimal ingredients—or make your own to control oils and salt.

7. Popcorn kernels

A wholesome, fiber-rich snack when popped in healthy oils or an air popper. Add herbs for extra flavor.

8. Pasta sauce

Glass jars or BPA-free cans of marinara, pesto, and tomato sauces offer ready-made options for grains, legumes, and proteins.

9. Nuts and nut butter

Stock raw or roasted almonds, walnuts, cashews, pistachios, hazelnuts, and their respective nut butters. Great for protein, healthy fats, and energy.

10. Canned chowder

Clam or fish-based chowders provide warmth and protein—just heat and serve.

11. Mayonnaise (shelf-stable versions)

Useful for sandwiches and salad dressings. Look for avocado oil-based or eggless mayo for better shelf life and healthier fat profiles.

12. Jelly & fruit preserves

Choose low-sugar or fruit-only options. They go well with nut butters, oat bars, or even as sweeteners in baked goods.

13. Canned chili

Look for bean-based, organic versions with minimal preservatives and no added sugar.

14. Iced tea (sugar-free)

Keep decaffeinated or herbal options like hibiscus or green iced tea blends in your pantry. These hydrate and provide antioxidants.

15. Bread-making ingredients

Essential for baking: bread flour, yeast, salt, sugar, baking powder, baking soda, and powdered eggs or milk.

16. Canned beans

Include black, kidney, navy, cannellini, pinto, and garbanzo beans. High in fiber, protein, and iron.

17. Hard candies

Useful not only for enjoyment but also to soothe dry throats or restore blood sugar levels during fatigue.

18. Crackers

Opt for whole grain or seed-based varieties. Pair them with nut butters, cheeses, or spreads.

19. Healthy cooking oils

Stock coconut oil, avocado oil, olive oil, and ghee. They are shelf-stable, versatile, and rich in good fats.

20. Canned fish

Include tuna, sardines, mackerel, and salmon. These provide omega-3s, protein, and essential vitamins.

21. Cookies

Buy whole grain or protein-enriched varieties, or make your own with oats, seeds, and dark chocolate.

22. Dark chocolate

A great source of antioxidants and magnesium. Store in cool, dry areas and use it for energy, baking, or morale-boosting!

23. Canned vegetables

Keep a rotation of corn, peas, green beans, spinach, carrots, and tomatoes. Use them in stews, stir-fries, or casseroles.

24. Canned soups

Look for organic, low-sodium, and high-protein options. Soups are great base meals or side dishes.

25. Canned meats

Include chicken, beef, turkey, or pulled pork. These provide protein-rich meals without needing refrigeration.

26. Canned fruits

Get pineapple, peaches, pears, and mixed fruits in natural juices—not syrup—for a vitamin boost and variety.

27. Breakfast cereals

Choose whole-grain cereals fortified with vitamins and minerals. Excellent for quick meals or snacks.

Additional recommended items

1. Powdered eggs – Ideal for baking or scrambled meals. Long shelf life and excellent protein source.

2. Dried fruit – Apricots, raisins, mango, apple chips. Great in bars, cereals, or as snacks.

3. Shelf-stable plant milks – Almond, oat, soy, or rice milk in tetrapacks.

4. Dehydrated soups or bouillon cubes – To flavor meals or rehydrate with beans, grains, or veggies.

5. Shelf-stable cheese – Hard cheeses (like Parmesan) or waxed cheese can last a long time unrefrigerated.

6. Vinegar & salt – For flavor, preservation, and cleaning purposes.

7. Honey & maple syrup – Natural sweeteners that don't expire.

8. Multivitamins – A practical backup if fresh produce becomes limited.

Final tips

- Rotate items frequently and check expiration dates.

- Store food in cool, dark, dry places.

- Label and organize your pantry with dates and categories.

- Keep an emergency manual can opener.

- Water is essential: store potable water and purification tablets if possible.

You now have a detailed, holistic guide to emergency food planning. This chapter—and the entire book—aims to empower you to face challenges with confidence, nutrition, and creativity.

Coming up: your printable survival food checklist!

Emergency grocery list for long-term storage

Dry staples

- White rice / Brown rice
    - Spaghetti / Macaroni / Pasta
    - Potato flakes
    - Oats (regular or instant)
    - Pancake mix or ingredients (flour, baking powder, etc.)
    - Bread ingredients (flour, salt, sugar, oil, yeast)
    - Breakfast cereals (fortified with vitamins or fruits)

Proteins & legumes

- Canned beans (black, pinto, great northern, etc.)
    - Canned chili
    - Canned fish (tuna, sardines, salmon, etc.)
    - Canned meats (chicken, beef, SPAM, etc.)
    - Eggs (fresh or powdered)
    - Protein powder
    - Nuts (almonds, walnuts, pistachios, etc.)
    - Nut butters (peanut butter, almond butter)

Fruits & vegetables

- Canned fruits (peaches, pineapples, fruit cocktails)
    - Canned vegetables (corn, green beans, peas, etc.)
    - Dried fruit (raisins, cranberries, apricots, etc.)

Snacks

- Granola

- Cookies
- Pretzels (unsalted preferred)
- Crackers
- Chocolates (dark chocolate preferred)
- Hard candies
- Potato chips
- Popcorn kernels

Beverages

- Sweetened powdered drink mix (natural sweeteners)
    - Berry drink mix
    - Cocoa mix / Cacao powder
    - Green tea / Iced tea
    - Pre-mixed canned drinks
    - Apple cider vinegar

Oils & condiments

- Coconut oil / Avocado oil / Olive oil / Butter / Lard
    - Mayonnaise
    - Jelly / Jam
    - Seasonings & dried herbs (oregano, garlic powder, cumin, etc.)
    - Salt and sugar

Supplements & superfoods

- Multivitamins
    - Vitamin C powder / Camu Camu powder
    - Digestive enzymes
    - Chlorella / Spirulina
    - Fiber powder (psyllium husk, bran, etc.)
    - Liquid minerals (magnesium, selenium, potassium)
    - Fish oil

- Water kefir grains

Seeds & add-ins

- Flaxseeds
  - Chia seeds
  - Hemp seeds
  - Sesame seeds
  - Almond seeds

Soups & prepared meals

- Canned soups (vegetable, chicken noodle, lentil, etc.)
  - Canned chowder (clam, corn, etc.)

Conclusion

C ongratulations on reaching the final chapter of this guide — a true act of foresight and self-care.

Your willingness to prepare not only speaks to your intelligence, but to your resilience. You've taken the crucial first step: awareness. And while knowledge is powerful, it is action that transforms lives. This book was written not just to inform, but to equip you to thrive — even in the most uncertain of times.

Emergencies do not announce themselves. They show up as power outages, closed stores, flooded roads, viral outbreaks, rising inflation, or geopolitical instability. And often, they arrive when we're least ready. But imagine facing such a moment with calm, confidence, and control — because you already knew what to do, what to eat, and how to care for yourself and your loved ones. That's the gift of preparedness.

You now understand:

- How nutrition is not just about survival, but about sustained health and energy

- How to build a long-lasting, balanced, and versatile food stockpile

- How to maintain proper digestion, support your immune system, and meet your family's diverse needs

- How to create simple, nutritious meals that comfort the body and calm the mind

But I urge you — do not let this book become another thing you meant to do someday. Emergencies are not scheduled. That's why preparation begins now. Start small if needed: one pantry shelf, one food category, one weekend shopping trip at a time.

Here's how to start today:

- Print or copy the food lists and create a weekly shopping plan

- Clear space in your pantry and freezer to accommodate your essentials

- Begin learning a few easy survival recipes using the items you've stored

- Teach your children or loved ones where supplies are, how to use them, and why it matters

- Rotate supplies every few months so nothing goes to waste

- Make a checklist of what you've stored, and add to it over time

This isn't about panic. It's about peace of mind. Having a well-thought-out food strategy means one less thing to worry about when the world becomes uncertain. It's about reclaiming control — not by reacting to chaos, but by calmly preparing for it in advance.

Let this book be your companion — not just in times of trouble, but in moments of growth.Use it to teach, to plan, to inspire healthier habits in daily life. Because what we do in ordinary times shapes how we survive extraordinary ones.

Whether you're a parent, caregiver, individual living alone, or someone responsible for others — your readiness matters. Your ability to nourish, heal, and sustain yourself is a gift not just for you, but for your entire household, community, and future.

The most powerful preparations begin quietly: one jar, one list, one choice at a time.

So go ahead. Fill your pantry with wisdom, your shelves with nourishment, and your heart with confidence. You're ready — more ready than most. Stay curious, stay compassionate, and above all, stay prepared.

You've got this.Now go and protect what matters most — one meal, one step, one plan at a time.

About the author

Dr. Lucy Coleman is a passionate advocate for health, longevity, and human empowerment. As a medical doctor, researcher, and bestselling author of over 50 books, she has dedicated her life to sharing practical, science-based knowledge that helps people thrive — not just survive.

Through her groundbreaking work in integrative and regenerative medicine, Dr. Coleman has supported thousands of individuals in reclaiming their well-being through smarter nutrition, lifestyle changes, and mental resilience. She is also the founder of , a global wellness platform designed to guide individuals toward greater vitality and personal strength.

In this essential guide to Survival Foods, Dr. Coleman combines her expertise in health and medicine with real-world strategies to help families prepare for emergencies. Whether facing pandemics, lockdowns, natural disasters, or economic challenges, her approach empowers readers to build confidence and stability through food preparedness. Together with her companion guides for surviving viral outbreaks and building strong immune defenses, this book offers a life-saving resource for anyone who wants to be truly ready for the unexpected.

Her mission is simple: to help you take back control of your health and your future — one informed choice at a time.

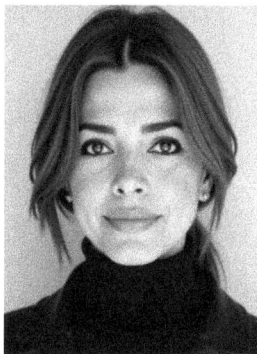

www.ingramcontent.com/pod-product-compliance
Lightning Source LLC
Chambersburg PA
CBHW060522280326
41933CB00014B/3068